A Guide To Gastro-oesophageal Reflux Disease

JS de Caestecker
Glenfield Hospital
Leicester, UK

JJ Misiewicz
Central Middlesex Hospital
London, UK

SCIENCE PRESS

British Library Cataloguing-in-Publication Data

A catalogue record for this book is available from the British Library.

ISBN: 1-85873-000-7

Sponsorship of this copy by Astra Pharmaceuticals Ltd does not imply the sponsor's agreement or otherwise with the views expressed herein.

Although every effort has been made to ensure that drug doses and other information are presented accurately in this publication, the ultimate responsibility rests with the prescribing physician. Neither the publishers nor the authors can be held responsible for errors or for any consequences arising from the use of the information contained herein. Any product mentioned in this publication should be used in accordance with the prescribing information prepared by the manufacturers. No claims or endorsements are made for any drug or compound at present under clinical investigation.

Project editors: Sara Churchill and Alison Taylor
Illustrator: Daniel Simmons
Production: Rebecca Spencer
Printed in Italy by Offset Print Veneta s.r.l.

Contents

Author biographies

John de Caestecker is Consultant Gastroenterologist at Glenfield Hospital, Leicester. He qualified at Cambridge University and the Middlesex Hospital, and acquired a continuing clinical and research interest in oesophageal motility disorders, non-cardiac chest pain and gastro-oesophageal reflux disease during training in Edinburgh.

George Misiewicz is a Consultant Physician and Joint Director of the Department of Gastroenterology at the Central Middlesex Hospital. His main areas of research in gastroenterology are disorders connected with acid/pepsin and *Helicobacter pylori*, and problems of gastrointestinal motility with reference to irritable bowel syndrome. He is the editor of the European Journal of Gastroenterology and Hepatology and a member of the External Scientific Staff, Medical Research Council.

A guide to gastro-oesophageal reflux disease

Gastro-oesophageal reflux disease (GORD) is probably the most common condition giving rise to dyspeptic symptoms in affluent societies today. This is true for both general practice and hospital-based gastroenterology, although different spectra of the disorder are found. Recent advances in diagnosis have brought recognition that the range of disease presentation is wide and varied. Although simple treatments are effective in many sufferers, therapeutic advances and a growing understanding of the natural history of the disorder are making it possible to provide effective medical treatment for most patients.

The concept of 'peptic oesophagitis', that is, distal oesophageal inflammation and ulceration related to reflux of gastric contents, was originally proposed approximately 60 years ago. Some 20 years later the essential abnormality was believed to be a hiatus hernia; for many non-medics and even some doctors, reflux symptoms and 'hiatus hernia' are still felt to be virtually synonymous, although this is now known not to be the case. The 1960s saw a growing understanding of the central role of an incompetent lower oesophageal sphincter leading to the present concept of GORD as a disease of multifactorial aetiology.

It is now recognised that GORD is a spectrum of related clinical disorders that ranges from patients with only symptomatic reflux to those with tissue damage. This concept has therapeutic implications: for some patients symptomatic relief will be sufficient whereas others will require healing of tissue damage and prevention of relapse.

Advances in pharmacological control of gastric output of acid and, to a lesser extent, in the control of upper-gut motility are having a major impact on the disease. The purpose of this book is to put these advances in knowledge into perspective in order to translate them into appropriate and effective treatment.

J S de Caestecker and J J Misiewicz

Terminology and definitions

Gastro-oesophageal reflux — the entry of gastric contents into the oesophagus. A degree of reflux occurs in everyone, but it becomes pathological when either symptoms or complications ensue.

Gastro-oesophageal reflux disease (GORD) — the term used to embrace all aspects of a condition now recognized to constitute a continuous spectrum of different but related clinical disorders. At one end of the spectrum are patients with 'symptomatic reflux', i.e. reflux that may be close to normal in terms of quantity but that produces troublesome symptoms like heartburn. The major abnormality in these individuals is a sensitive oesophageal mucosa. At the other end are patients with tissue damage resulting from the action of refluxate on the oesophageal mucosa. Some will have symptoms similar to symptomatic reflux, but others will have complications such as dysphagia or bleeding.

Hiatus hernia — an anatomical derangement caused by the herniation of the cardia and a portion of stomach through the diaphragmatic hiatus. The hernia may reduce spontaneously and is often present without abnormal reflux. Conversely, not all patients with abnormal gastro-oesophageal reflux have a hiatus hernia. This term is not a synonym for gastro-oesophageal reflux.

Oesophagitis — the mucosal damage that may result from GORD. It does not necessarily occur and should not be regarded as synonymous with GORD.

Barrett's oesophagus — the presence of gastric-type epithelium more than 3cm above the lower oesophageal sphincter.

1. Clinical presentation of GORD

Classic symptoms

Heartburn is a burning retrosternal discomfort extending anywhere from the epigastrium to the throat. It characteristically occurs after eating, bending or lying flat. It may also occur during vigorous exercise, particularly if undertaken after a meal.

Acid regurgitation or **acid brash** is the sensation of sour-tasting gastric contents reaching the pharynx. It occurs after the same manoeuvres that provoke heartburn and both may occur simultaneously.

Associated symptoms may include:

- **waterbrash** — the production of copious tasteless saliva, usually in response to heartburn.

- **belching** — a non-specific symptom which may also result from a variety of other conditions producing discomfort in the chest or upper abdomen.

- **odynophagia** — pain on swallowing, particularly of hot liquids or food. This is more common in the presence of oesophagitis.

The first two symptoms, heartburn and acid regurgitation, are a reliable guide to the diagnosis of GORD if they are the patient's chief complaint.

Atypical symptoms

Atypical symptoms are a reasonably common mode of presentation of GORD, at least in hospital practice, where they may account for between a third to one half of all patients diagnosed as having this condition. Symptoms include:

- non-specific upper abdominal pain.
- nausea and vomiting.
- non-specific chest pain, which may radiate to the back.
- angina-like chest pain, with the characteristic pattern of radiation to

the left arm and neck or jaw. In this case, the pain often occurs at rest or at night and may be long lasting. Any relationship to exercise is often highly variable. Provocation of pain by food or posture, or the presence of other oesophageal symptoms, are a clue.

- globus, though recent evidence has cast doubt on whether this is truly related to reflux.

- chest problems, including nocturnal wheezing or coughing and recurrent pneumonia, are rarely caused by gastro-oesophageal reflux.

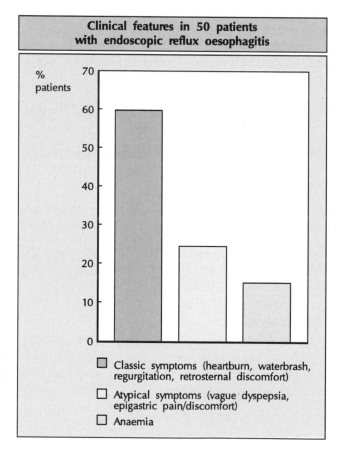

Clinical features in 50 patients with endoscopic oesophagitis. Adapted by permission from Heading RC, *et al.*: Long-term management of reflux patients. In Cimetidine in the 1980's, edited by JH Baron. Edinburgh:Churchill Livingstone 1981, pp172–180.

Reflux in infancy

The most common symptoms in this age group are anaemia, regurgitation and recurrent chest infections, the former arising from bleeding and the latter from aspiration. Some regurgitation occurs physiologically anyway in the first six months of life but these symptoms of GORD normally resolve with time. The tendency for spontaneous improvement in paediatric reflux over the first two years of life means that, except in the most severe cases, medical treatment is preferred. There is some evidence that some cases of cot death result from gastro-oesophageal reflux.

Symptoms suggesting complications

Dysphagia is the sensation of food 'sticking' anywhere between the throat and epigastrium. This characteristically signals the development of a stricture, but can also occur in GORD in the absence of this. In benign stricture, dysphagia is usually slowly progressive and, at least in the early stages, mainly occurs only with solids.

Dysphagia, particularly in older men, can be the first sign of oesophageal adenocarcinoma, a recognized complication of Barrett's oesophagus in long-standing GORD. Weight loss and anorexia may also be evident, if the tumour is advanced. Other symptoms could include odynophagia or, if the tumour has invaded the mediastinum, unremitting pain, which can radiate to the back.

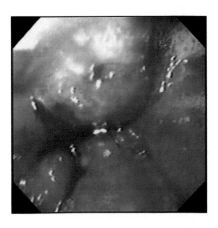

Oesophageal adenocarcinoma in a Barrett's oesophagus.

CLINICAL PRESENTATION OF GORD

Symptoms produced by GORD	
Classic symptoms	Heartburn, pharyngeal regurgitation of gastric contents, odynophagia
Atypical symptoms	Vague dyspepsia, epigastric pain, non-cardiac chest pain
Symptoms due to complications	Dysphagia, symptoms of acute or chronic blood loss
Respiratory symptoms	Hoarseness, cough, asthma

Haematemesis and melaena may occur, especially in elderly and bed-bound patients who often develop particularly severe oesophagitis. Life threatening haemorrhage is unusual, except when acute bleeding arises from a Barrett's ulcer (chronic peptic ulcer within a Barrett's oesophagus).

Symptoms of anaemia may arise from chronic bleeding from oesophagitis. Unless the oesophagitis is severe, it is mandatory to investigate for other potential sources of gastrointestinal blood loss, for example, a colonic neoplasm.

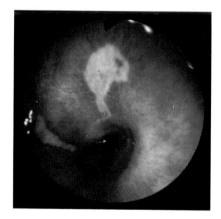

Barrett's ulcer in the columnar segment. Published by permission of GNJ Tytgat, Academic Medical Centre, Amsterdam, The Netherlands. © Astra 1993.

2. An approach to diagnosis

Comparisons with long-term pH monitoring have indicated that the typical symptoms of heartburn with postprandial and postural provocation and acid regurgitation are highly specific for the diagnosis of GORD. Unfortunately these symptoms are not very sensitive (*see Appendix III*). In patients under the age of 45 years, if symptoms are typical, especially if long-standing, the diagnosis can be made without further investigation and treatment started.

Older patients, especially if the history is recent, must be investigated. Other symptoms which prompt early investigation include dysphagia, vomiting and weight loss. The former two symptoms, if long-standing and non-progressive, may not indicate other serious disease. The best initial investigation is endoscopy because the most important diagnosis to be excluded in the above two groups is oesophagogastric malig-

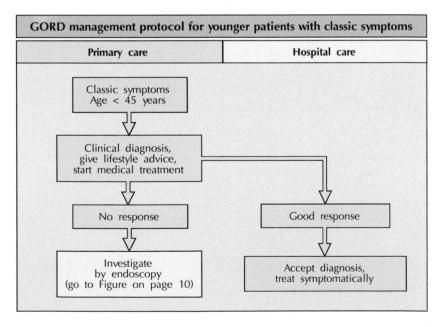

GORD management protocol for younger patients with classic symptoms

Primary care	Hospital care

Classic symptoms
Age < 45 years

Clinical diagnosis,
give lifestyle advice,
start medical treatment

No response

Good response

Investigate
by endoscopy
(go to Figure on page 10)

Accept diagnosis,
treat symptomatically

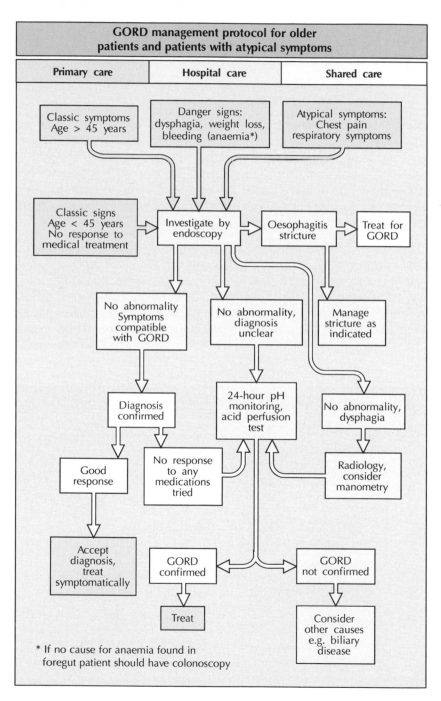

GORD management protocol for older patients and patients with atypical symptoms

Primary care	Hospital care	Shared care

Classic symptoms
Age > 45 years

Danger signs:
dysphagia, weight loss,
bleeding (anaemia*)

Atypical symptoms:
Chest pain
respiratory symptoms

Classic signs
Age < 45 years
No response to
medical treatment

Investigate by
endoscopy

Oesophagitis
stricture

Treat for
GORD

No abnormality
Symptoms
compatible
with GORD

No abnormality,
diagnosis
unclear

Manage
stricture as
indicated

Diagnosis
confirmed

24-hour pH
monitoring,
acid perfusion
test

No abnormality,
dysphagia

Good
response

No response
to any
medications
tried

Radiology,
consider
manometry

Accept
diagnosis,
treat
symptomatically

GORD
confirmed

GORD
not confirmed

Treat

Consider
other causes
e.g. biliary
disease

* If no cause for anaemia found in
foregut patient should have colonoscopy

nancy. However, double-contrast barium radiology, if more readily available, is a good alternative.

Patients with typical symptoms or with non-specific dyspepsia who fail to respond to antacids or acid-lowering agents such as proton pump inhibitors or H_2-receptor antagonists should be investigated, initially by endoscopy. A barium swallow, carefully performed, is also valuable. If the diagnosis is still not clear and GORD is possible, an acid perfusion test may help to indicate whether the pain has an oesophageal origin. If available, prolonged oesophageal pH monitoring is probably the most useful diagnostic test.

Patients with oesophagitis who have a poor symptomatic response to maximal therapy with proton pump inhibitors must likewise be investigated (*see later*) although their oesophagitis may have resolved. These people should be investigated by pH monitoring while remaining on treatment, because a few patients fail to suppress gastric acid secretion even with large doses of omeprazole [1]. If pH monitoring is negative, another diagnosis should be considered.

Details of various investigative techniques are given at the end of the book.

AN APPROACH TO DIAGNOSIS

3. Differential diagnosis

Cardiac disease

Some patients with ischaemic heart disease may present with atypical chest pain, sometimes of a burning quality. The clue is usually in a relationship between pain and exercise and subsequent relief by rest.

Patients with angina may experience symptoms which are provoked by meals or bending. Others, with severe coronary artery disease, have decubitus angina, waking them at night. Both these symptoms can of course also occur in GORD.

In approximately one fifth of patients admitted to hospital with acute chest pain the cause is oesophageal [2]. The differentiation from GORD in any of these situations may not be straightforward.

GORD is common in the very patients in whom coronary artery disease frequently occurs and an interaction is possible. For example, oesophageal acid exposure may provoke angina with ischaemic ECG changes in patients with coronary artery disease and patients may be unable to differentiate oesophageal from anginal pain. Because many drugs used to treat angina can provoke reflux (e.g. nitrates and calcium channel antagonists) the potential for interaction can be readily appreciated.

Conversely, some patients with oesophageal disease may have symptoms very similar to cardiac angina. Reflux can occur on exertion and acid-induced pain may have the same characteristics and radiation as cardiac pain. There may be clues in the history to suggest an oesophageal rather than cardiac origin:

- pain with an inconstant relation to exercise.
- pain lasting for hours after exercise.
- pain occurring after meals or on bending, particularly if associated with other oesophageal symptoms.
- a constant background pain with exacerbation after meals or exercise.

Cardiac disease and gastro-oesophageal reflux disease	
• Angina may have features similar to heartburn	• Some patients with apparent cardiac pain in fact have oesophageal disease
• Anti-anginal drug therapy may provoke reflux	• Gastro-oesophageal acid reflux may either mimic angina or provoke angina with ECG changes in patients with ischaemic heart disease

Gastro-oesophageal reflux is known to be the most common treatable cause of oesophageal pain mimicking cardiac pain. Usually, however, patients presenting in this fashion should have a cardiological work-up (which may or may not include coronary angiography, depending on the degree of suspicion) before the oesophagus is studied.

Pulmonary disease

In a few patients recurrent aspiration pneumonia is secondary to reflux and in others asthma is triggered by reflux. Diagnosis in the former may be facilitated by scintigraphy the morning after drinking fluid labelled with a radio-isotope, which may then be seen in the lungs. The latter is most easily diagnosed by oesophageal pH monitoring, especially overnight, to establish a correlation between reflux and wheezing episodes.

It is well known that patients with chronic obstructive airways disease have a higher than expected prevalence of gastro-oesophageal reflux; abnormal amounts of reflux are present in some 60–80% of these patients when investigated by pH monitoring [3]. In most cases the reflux is probably secondary to the airways obstruction (possibly arising from stress-induced reflux caused by coughing, medication such as beta-agonists and methyl xanthines, which impair lower oesophageal sphincter pressure, or impaired function of the flattened diaphragm). It is still contentious whether this reflux is important in the respiratory disease. Patients with recurrent pneumonia and troublesome nocturnal asthma responding poorly to medication should be referred for oesophageal investigation, particularly if they have reflux symptoms.

Other gastro-intestinal disorders

Patients who have a duodenal ulcer or irritable bowel syndrome have a higher than expected incidence of GORD. In some cases reflux dominates the symptoms. In patients with irritable bowel syndrome, the problem is an acid-sensitive oesophagus, whereas approximately 20–30% of patients with a duodenal ulcer have oesophagitis [4]. Duodenal ulcer may present with chest, rather than epigastric pain.

Oesophageal carcinoma and motility disorders may produce chest pain resembling heartburn, but this symptom is usually overshadowed by dysphagia and odynophagia.

Biliary colic occasionally presents with chest, rather than epigastric or right upper quadrant pain, although this is more likely to be confused with cardiac than with oesophageal disease.

4. Medical treatment

GORD is a condition characterized by disordered oesophagogastric motility and thus impaired clearance of refluxed acid. Unfortunately, treatment aimed at correcting underlying motility disorders has so far been only partially successful. However, an appreciation of the main pathogenic mechanisms of the disease and of its spectrum has been gained through motility studies and has allowed informed and appropriate management. The availability of more effective suppressants of gastric acid secretion, such as proton pump inhibitors, has made highly successful therapy possible.

General measures

The measures listed over the page are an essential part of good management and must underpin drug treatment.

Effects of specific foods in GORD			
Food	Lower oesophageal sphincter pressure	Oesophageal receptor stimulation	Other effects
Chocolate	Decreased		Decreased gastric emptying
Fats	Decreased		Decreased gastric emptying
Coffee	Slightly decreased		Increased gastric acid secretion
Orange/ tomato juice		Stimulated	
Alcohol	Decreased	Stimulated	Impaired oesophageal motility
Peppermint	Decreased		

Weight loss is well known to diminish symptoms, even to the point of dispensing with drug treatment in some cases. Although weight loss has not been formally investigated, it presumably works simply by reducing intra-abdominal pressure. The wearing of belts and tight clothing is discouraged for the same reason.

Avoidance of certain foods: some, such as fatty food (probably in part through release of cholecystokinin), coffee and alcohol are known to decrease lower oesophageal sphincter pressure. Others, such as onions, citrus fruits, tomato and other fruit juices directly stimulate an inflamed or sensitized oesophageal mucosa.

Eating habits: Large meals distend the stomach and give rise to decreased lower oesophageal sphincter tone and a higher rate of transient sphincter relaxations during which reflux may occur. The main meal of the day is often in the evening and most reflux occurs following this event. This is particularly so if the meal is taken shortly before retiring to bed, when oesophageal clearance mechanisms are impaired. It is advisable, therefore, for patients to eat smaller, evenly spaced, meals during the day and avoid eating (or having a 'nightcap') in the three hours before retiring to bed.

Smoking has been shown to increase the frequency of reflux episodes and should be discouraged. However, this measure may be less helpful than weight reduction.

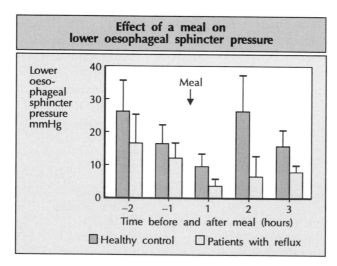

Effect of a meal on lower oesophageal sphincter pressure

Lower oesophageal sphincter pressure mmHg

Time before and after meal (hours)

☐ Healthy control   ☐ Patients with reflux

Lower oesophageal sphincter pressure two hours before and three hours after a meal. Published by permission from Baldi F, *et al.* Gut 1985, 26:336–341.

Posture: Propping up the head of the bed on 6 inch wooden blocks, alone or in association with acid suppression, has been shown in a controlled clinical trial to hasten resolution of symptoms and healing of oesophagitis. A foam wedge under the mattress is also effective, but using extra pillows does not seem to be. These measures improve oesophageal clearance of refluxed gastric acid during sleep. They are indicated even in the absence of nocturnal symptoms because nocturnal acid exposure may sensitize oesophageal pain receptors making heartburn more likely during the day.

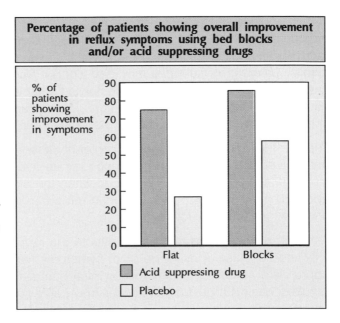

Percentage of patients showing overall improvement in reflux symptoms using bed blocks and/or acid suppressing drugs

% of patients showing improvement in symptoms

Effect of using bed blocks on the symptoms of oesophagitis with or without the use of an acid suppressing drug. Adapted by permission from Harvey RF, *et al.* Lancet 1987, i:1200–1203. © The Lancet, 1987.

MEDICAL TREATMENT

The patient must be advised to avoid bending or stooping whenever possible.

Antacids and alginates

No controlled clinical trial has shown superiority of antacids over placebo in the relief of reflux symptoms. This is at variance with the experience of the majority of sufferers, many of whom use them without ever consulting a doctor. Support for this common experience comes from one American study, in which individuals using antacids on a daily basis for heartburn were recruited by advertisement. In a month-long controlled trial, 30 of 33 people correctly differentiated the antacid from placebo [5].

Only three of eight controlled trials with alginates have shown a significant improvement over placebo. This is again at variance with clinical use. It should be noted that alginates may be used ineffectively if the mechanism of action is not appreciated [6].

These compounds work through a floating raft of alginate formed with carbon dioxide liberated by the action of gastric acid on sodium bicarbonate in the mixture. Intercountry differences in formulation affect raft strength and this could be one reason for some of the negative trial results. Different formulations may also contain variable (but small) amounts of aluminium/magnesium-containing antacids, but these only neutralize a trivial amount of gastric acid. The efficacy is more related to the mechanical barrier function of the alginate raft.

The raft should float on top of gastric contents, although between meals the contents are small in volume and the alginate is rapidly lost from the stomach. Maximum effect is produced when the alginates are given about 30 minutes after meals, when the raft will form above the food and be emptied more slowly.

Although neither group of drugs is effective in healing oesophagitis, they are very useful in the relief of symptoms. Antacids are most appropriately used for relief of mild or infrequent symptoms on an 'as required' basis. Large, frequent doses may partially neutralize gastric acid, but this is impractical and may lead to side effects, such as diarrhoea. Alginates used in-between meals on an 'as required' basis probably act as simple antacids, because their raft effect will be redundant in the absence of food. They are best used regularly after meals and before bed for the reasons given earlier.

Side effects of these compounds include constipation (aluminium/calcium salts), diarrhoea (magnesium salts), hypernatraemia or, very rarely, metabolic alkalosis (sodium bicarbonate) and hypercalcaemia. Patients requiring sodium restriction (for example, in heart failure or cirrhosis of the liver with ascites) should not be given sodium-containing compounds.

Flotation and selective retention of an alginate compared with a conventional antacid in the gastric fundus

Aluminium-hydroxide-magnesium oxide suspension

Sodium-alginate, sodium bicarbonate antireflux agent

Flotation and selective retention of an alginate in the fundus compared with a conventional antacid. Reprinted with permission from Washington N, Handbook of Antacids and anti-reflux agents, © CRC Press, Boca Raton, Florida, USA. 1991.

Acid-suppressing agents

Although a decrease in the aggressive factors in gastric juice renders refluxate less noxious, reflux may still occur because the underlying mechanisms which permit this event remain unaffected.

In general, the greater the ability of a drug to inhibit acid production, the greater its efficacy in the treatment of GORD. Drugs with a longer duration of action are also advantageous in this condition, because symptom relief and healing of oesophagitis are achieved faster and in a greater proportion of patients if 24-hour acid suppression is obtained. This is because the severity of the disorder is related to the total acid exposure of the oesophageal mucosa. Nocturnal acid inhibition, so effective in the treatment of peptic ulcer disease, is less impressive in GORD.

MEDICAL TREATMENT

21

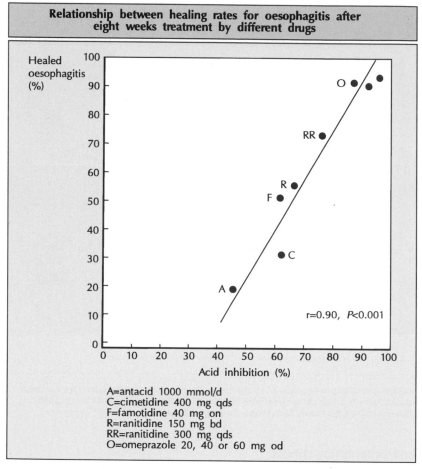

Relationship between healing rates for oesophagitis after eight weeks treatment by different drugs

Healed oesophagitis (%)

Acid inhibition (%)

r=0.90, P<0.001

A=antacid 1000 mmol/d
C=cimetidine 400 mg qds
F=famotidine 40 mg on
R=ranitidine 150 mg bd
RR=ranitidine 300 mg qds
O=omeprazole 20, 40 or 60 mg od

Relationship between healing rates for oesophagitis and gastric acid suppression after eight weeks treatment with different drugs. Reprinted from High doses of ranitidine in patients with reflux oesophagitis by Jansen JBMJ and Lamers CBHW from Scand J Gastroenterol 1990, 25(Suppl):42–46, by permisssion of Scandinavian University Press.

H₂-receptor antagonists

H2-receptor antagonists were the first class of drug able to achieve clinically useful inhibition of acid output, but, although a considerable advance in reflux treatment, they had greatest impact in the treatment of peptic ulcer. This is probably because a much greater degree of acid suppression is needed for the successful treatment of GORD.

Symptom control is achieved in approximately 80% of patients after six–eight weeks of treatment but it may take up to six weeks before the maximum effect is attained. Larger and more frequent doses may have a more complete and rapid effect (e.g., cimetidine 800 mg four times daily or ranitidine 150 mg four times daily) but, as these are both expensive and cumbersome to use, compliance may be poor.

The ability of H_2-receptor antagonists to heal oesophagitis depends on the initial grade of oesophagitis and the dose and frequency of administration of the H_2-receptor antagonist. Overall, the healing rate (complete healing as assessed by endoscopy) is about 50% after six–eight weeks treatment, but is much better for Grade I (80% or more healed) than for more severe oesophagitis (20–30% healed).

The results are improved by prolonging the period of treatment to three or more months, although this is an expensive option, and by increasing the frequency and size of the dose.

Patients who fail to respond to H_2-receptor antagonists may do so because the drugs fail to adequately suppress basal or stimulated gastric acid output. Consequently, the noxious nature of refluxed gastric acid is little affected in these individuals.

H_2-receptor antagonists are most appropriately used in patients whose symptoms fail to respond to general measures and antacids, or alginates. In general, they are most useful for the treatment of reflux in patients without oesophagitis or those with mild forms (grades I and II). Recommended starting doses are cimetidine 400 mg four times daily or ranitidine 150 mg twice daily with the option of increasing the dose and frequency of administration (cimetidine 800mg four times daily or ranitidine 150 mg four times daily) or changing to a more longer-acting drug (e.g. famotidine 20–40 mg twice daily). Nocturnal dosing alone is usually less effective, but may be helpful in patients in whom symptoms occur principally at night.

Side effects are unusual and include rashes, confusion in the elderly, transient liver enzyme elevations and hyperprolactinaemia leading to gynaecomastia and galactorrhoea. These drugs may also result in inhibition of the liver cytochrome P_{450} group of microsomal mixed function oxidases responsible for metabolism of drugs such as phenytoin, warfarin and theophylline which results in an increase in their serum levels. This latter effect is particularly found with cimetidine. In practice, these side effects are rarely of clinical significance but the

MEDICAL TREATMENT

latter drug interactions in particular should be born in mind. The P_{450} oxidase inhibition does, however, seem to occur less frequently with newer H_2-receptor antagonists such as famotidine.

Proton pump inhibitors

Most of the available evidence for this class of drugs concerns omeprazole which produces a specific dose-dependent inhibition of the gastric proton pump (H^+/K^+ ATPase) in the parietal cell, the final common pathway of gastric acid production. It is therefore highly effective in relieving symptoms and healing all grades of oesophagitis [7,8]. A daily dose of omeprazole 20 mg results in over 80% healing at eight weeks in the treatment of mild oesophagitis [8]. Omeprazole 40 mg daily used to treat severe oesophagitis results in over 63% healing at four weeks and 90% healing at 12 weeks [9]. These healing rates, particularly in severe cases, are a considerable improvement on the best results achievable with the H_2-receptor antagonists. Although comparable healing rates have sometimes been reported with high-dose H_2-receptor antagonist (e.g. ranitidine 300 mg four times daily), this option is relatively expensive and can lead to problems with compliance. Symptoms also respond faster with omeprazole than with the H_2-receptor antagonists [7,10], irrespective of the initial severity of symptoms. The ability of omeprazole to heal even 'resistant oesophagitis' (defined as unhealed after three months of treatment with standard/high-dose H_2-receptor antagonists), a situation which probably occurs in approximately 10–15% of patients with this disorder, is demonstrated by a recent study comparing omeprazole 40 mg daily with ranitidine 300 mg twice daily [9]. Treatment with omeprazole heals over 90% of patients after 12 weeks at a dose of 40 mg daily, compared with less than 50% of patients receiving ranitidine. Omeprazole is suitable for all grades of oesophagitis and is particularly effective in the treatment of severe (grades III and IV) or complicated oesophagitis.

Omeprazole is also very effective at healing peptic ulcers within Barrett's oesophagus and is more effective than ranitidine in relation to recurrence of strictures [11]. There do exist rare patients who are resistant to high doses of this drug, because gastric acid production is not totally suppressed.

Omeprazole is well tolerated; reported side effects include headache, rash and diarrhoea. Concerns have been raised that profound acid inhibition could cause benign carcinoid tumours due to increased

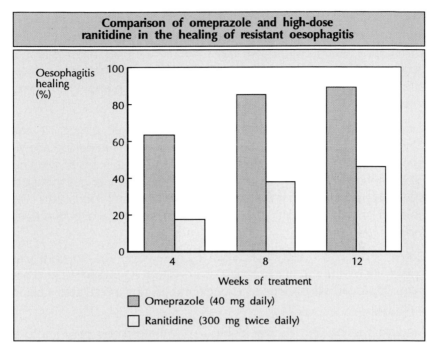

Comparison of omeprazole and high-dose ranitidine in the healing of resistant oesophagitis

Oesophagitis healing (%)

Weeks of treatment

☐ Omeprazole (40 mg daily)
☐ Ranitidine (300 mg twice daily)

Comparison of omeprazole and high-dose ranitidine in the healing of resistant oesophagitis. Published by permission from Blackwell Scientific Publications Limited. Lundell L, *et al.:* Aliment Pharmacol Therap 1990, 4:145–155.

gastrin levels. This is not supported by current evidence even in patients on very high doses of omeprazole for many years. Omeprazole inhibits the metabolism of warfarin and phenytoin, which necessitates monitoring of patients receiving these drugs.

Prokinetic agents

Metoclopramide, domperidone and cisapride are all related substituted benzamides.

Metoclopramide, the first compound in this class to be developed, is a derivative of procainamide with antidopaminergic actions and is active centrally (because it crosses the blood-brain barrier) and peripherally. It has a prokinetic effect on the gut by virtue of stimulating acetylcholine release from the myenteric plexus; it is also a weak 5-HT$_3$ (serotonin) antagonist. It has been shown to increase lower oesophageal sphincter pressure and to accelerate gastric emptying after a meal.

MEDICAL TREATMENT

Domperidone is a related compound which does not cross the blood–brain barrier and thus has peripheral effects only. It acts as a dopamine D_2-receptor antagonist. In this way it counters the inhibitory effect of dopamine on oesophagogastric motility. Although it has little clinical effect on distal oesophageal motility it does increase gastric emptying rate.

Cisapride has neither central nor antidopaminergic effects. It was developed as a specific prokinetic agent and acts by releasing acetylcholine from the gut myenteric plexus and possibly by stimulating presynaptic serotonin 5-HT_4 receptors. It increases lower oesophageal sphincter pressure, stimulates distal oesophageal peristalsis, increases gastric emptying rate and co-ordinates antral and duodenal motility.

Bethanechol is a direct cholinergic agonist which has no particular specificity for the gut. It increases lower oesophageal sphincter pressure, improves oesophageal acid clearance and stimulates gastric emptying.

Metoclopramide and domperidone 10 mg three times daily improve symptoms significantly better than placebo in most trials of their use in GORD. Most studies have involved metoclopramide, which is about as effective as the H_2-receptor antagonists in this respect. However, neither compound is effective in healing oesophagitis. The disadvantages of metoclopramide are the side effects arising from its central action; these include drowsiness and extrapyramidal side effects such as akathisia (restless legs), acute dystonias (such as torticollis or lockjaw) and Parkinsonism (particularly in the elderly). Tardive dyskinesia may occur in long-term therapy. These side effects are not a problem with domperidone. Both drugs are cheap and may be particularly useful where symptoms include other dyspeptic features such as nausea, vomiting, bloating or early satiety.

Bethanecol is similar in efficacy to metoclopramide, but is little used in the UK. Its main drawbacks stem from its lack of specificity, resulting in predictable side effects related to its muscarinic agonist activity. These include abdominal cramps, diarrhoea, urinary frequency or urgency and increased upper respiratory tract secretions.

Cisapride is the newest and most interesting of these compounds. Its effect on symptoms has been shown in controlled trials to be comparable to that of the H_2-receptor antagonists and it is the only prokinetic agent to have been shown to heal oesophagitis [12]. Like the H_2-receptor antagonists, it is most effective in milder grades (I and II) of oesophagitis. There is some evidence that combination with cimetidine is more effective than either drug separately. At a therapeutic dose of 10 mg three times daily it has few side effects, the most common are abdominal cramps and diarrhoea. Of particular interest is new evidence that maintenance cisapride may be effective in preventing relapse [13] (*see later*).

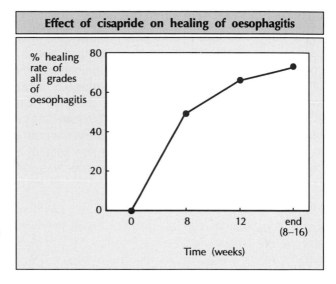

Effect of cisapride on healing of oesophagitis. Adapted by permission from Toussaint J, *et al.* Gut 1991, 32:1280–1285.

Other drugs

Mucosal protective drugs, such as sucralfate, carbenoxolone and bismuth salts, have similar oesophagitis healing rates to the H_2-receptor antagonists. Carbenoxolone is very little used now because it can produce severe side effects in the form of sodium retention, oedema, hypokalaemia and hypertension. Most of these compounds have not been studied extensively and it is unclear whether they may have an additive effect in combination with acid-suppressing drugs.

There is theoretical evidence to implicate prostaglandins as protective or as injurious to the oesophageal mucosa, depending on the damaging agent and the animal model. They are probably protective in humans as far as acid-induced damage is concerned. One study has suggested clinical benefit for a prostaglandin analogue, trimoprostil, in the treatment of GORD.

Selective antimuscarinic compounds, such as pirenzepine, have no adverse effect on distal oesophageal motility (unlike conventional anticholinergic agents) and are capable of suppressing gastric acid secretion. Clinical studies are few and inconclusive and so the usefulness of this group of drugs is uncertain.

Cost effectiveness of medical therapies

In the current climate of budgetary restriction in many national health care systems, considerations of cost effectiveness in prescribing are important. A number of studies have examined the cost effectiveness of omeprazole compared with the H_2-receptor antagonists in terms of symptom relief and healing. Findings from the USA [14] and the UK [15,16] have shown that when symptom relief and healing rates were used as end points, omeprazole was the more cost effective treatment in the short term compared with either ranitidine or cimetidine, despite being more expensive than the H_2- receptor antagonists on a dose-for-dose basis.

5. Surgical treatment

Indications for surgery are now fewer because medical treatments have improved. In adult patients with GORD they include:

- **Failure of response to vigorous medical treatment** (no longer common). As already indicated, on rare occasions patients fail to respond to even high doses of a proton pump inhibitor. The most compelling case for surgical treatment is continued marked regurgitation, perhaps despite the control of heartburn. These patients have a severe functional and mechanical defect at the cardia and complain of unrelenting regurgitation of gastric contents. This symptom is poorly controlled by medical treatment.

- **Severe complications**, particularly in younger (< 50 years old) patients. These may include non-healing peptic ulcer in a Barrett's oesophagus or benign stricture.

- **True alkaline reflux disease**, especially if complicated by severe oesophagitis which is difficult to treat medically. This condition is confined to patients with prior gastric surgery, particularly if cholecystectomy has already been done, and may be an indication for a biliary diversion procedure (e.g., Roux-en-Y conversion).

- **Pulmonary aspiration**, particularly in children.

- **Rapid relapse** on stopping medical treatment is no longer such an important indication because omeprazole can now be used for long periods in the more severe cases.

- **Non-compliance** with treatment is sometimes regarded as an indication for surgery. This is a difficult decision and it is hard to make a generalization about the value of surgery in these circumstances.

Types of operation

A large number of anti-reflux operations have been developed, reflecting the unsatisfactory results of any single procedure. The aim of most is to create an artificial mechanical buttress to the lower oesophageal sphincter mechanism. The first procedure used, hiatal repair, had a high recurrence and failure rate. The most popular procedure today is some form of fundoplication (a wrap of gastric fundus around the lower oesophagus). The most widely practised is a 360° wrap — the Nissen fundoplication. A partial wrap (such as the Belsey Mark IV) or a loose ('floppy') Nissen may be advantageous, if oesophageal peristalsis is grossly impaired, in order to avoid postoperative dysphagia. Some units have reported antireflux surgery performed through the laparoscope; although this is now feasible it is time consuming and long-term results are at present unknown.

Some years ago there was a spate of enthusiasm for the silicone ring, the Angelchik device, the advantages being speed and simplicity of operation. The ring is placed surgically below the diaphragm around the distal oesophagus. However, the occurrence of major complications (*see later*) have tempered enthusiasm for its use.

Oesophageal resection is only rarely indicated for severe complications such as unresponsive strictures. Additional procedures to lengthen the oesophagus, such as a Collis gastroplasty, or interposition of a length of jejunum or colon, may then be needed.

Results of surgery

Most modern operations (including the Angelchik prosthesis) control reflux disease in more than 80% of patients in the short term (1–2 years) but long-term follow-up (up to 10 years) has shown that the incidence of failure increases with time.

Early complications include all of those normally associated with abdominal surgery, for example, chest and wound infections and venous thromboembolism. Elderly, obese patients with cardiorespiratory disease are at high risk and surgery should be avoided in these individuals.

Dysphagia is common in the early postoperative period, occurring in up to 40% of individuals (particularly with the Angelchik device but also after Nissen fundoplication). This dysphagia is usually mild and transient, resolving after three months in most individuals. In a minority of people it may be severe enough to warrant reversal of the operation.

An inability to belch or vomit results in the '*gas bloat syndrome*' (gastric bloating and postprandial fullness) which may be aggravated by damage of the vagus nerve at operation, because the capacity of the stomach to relax during distension may be impaired. This complication is often persistent and may be disabling. Individuals who habitually swallow air and consequently belch a great deal are most likely to suffer from this troublesome complication. These people should avoid operations.

Vagus nerve damage may occasionally lead to *postoperative gastroparesis*.

Complications peculiar to the Angelchik prosthesis include migration of the device within the abdomen or chest, sudden total dysphagia arising from rotation or angulation, or erosion of the ring into the stomach, from which it may then be passed per rectum. This latter complication usually occurs several months after insertion of the prosthesis and is not accompanied by free perforation into the peritoneum. It occurs principally in patients who have another procedure done at the time of insertion of the device, such as a vagotomy.

Overall, major or minor complications occur in 25–40% of patients. Because some complications are persistent and may be as disabling as the reflux symptoms for which the operation was performed, the decision to operate should be taken carefully.

Reoperation for failed antireflux surgery

Failure may arise from the complications described or recurrent reflux. These patients should undergo oesophageal motility and pH studies and some individuals may need measurement of gastric emptying. A drainage procedure, such as a pyloroplasty, may be indicated in some cases. In patients with recurrent reflux, if reoperation is judged essential, the surgical options include revision of the fundoplication procedure (which may necessitate a thoracic or thoracoabdominal approach), vagotomy, antrectomy and Roux-en-Y bile diversion.

SURGICAL TREATMENT

6. Management summary

The aim of good management is accurate diagnosis followed by effective treatment. Treatment goals include relief of symptoms, resolution of complications and the prevention of relapse.

Symptom relief

Symptom relief is the main aim in most patients, including those presenting with typical symptoms in whom an initial diagnosis is based on history and examination and those whose diagnosis has been established by investigation. In order to obtain a satisfactory degree of symptom relief, as determined by the patient, an assessment of his/her quality of life will be required. Patients may be prepared to live with occasional symptoms which do not interfere with activities. This philosophy is appropriate even in patients with oesophagitis, if the degree of tissue damage is mild (grades I and II), because available follow-up studies indicate a low likelihood of both deterioration in the oesophagitis and the development of complications. Furthermore, the mortality from oesophagitis is very small, of the order of 0.1/100,000 per year, very much less than that from peptic ulcer.

All patients should be encouraged to adjust their lifestyle. The most important general measures are weight loss in obese patients and propping up the head of the bed at night, *even for people without nocturnal symptoms.* (The latter requires the use of bed blocks or a foam wedge because the use of additional pillows alone is ineffective in promoting oesophageal clearance). Smoking should also be discouraged.

Certain foods should be avoided especially if patients recognize them to provoke symptoms, for example, coffee and fruit juice. It is appropriate that the patient eats smaller meals at regular intervals and avoids eating three hours before bedtime (*see page 18*).

Drug therapy should be individually tailored to the patient's symptom type and frequency, keeping in mind possible adverse reactions and cost. There is no standard treatment suitable for all patients with reflux. For example, a patient with reflux symptoms and abdominal pain and intermittent diarrhoea arising from the irritable bowel syndrome might have the latter made worse by a prokinetic agent, whereas another with reflux symptoms and nausea, vomiting or early satiety might most appropriately be treated in this way.

Infrequent symptoms (once a week or less often), particularly if not severe, can be treated by antacids as needed. More frequent symptoms, particularly after meals, can initially be managed with regular postprandial alginates.

Patients who fail to respond to these simple measures may respond to cimetidine 400mg twice or three times daily, or to omeprazole 20mg daily. The latter may be preferable because, apart from providing rapid relief of symptoms in most patients, it is usually cheaper and more acceptable to patients than large doses of H_2-receptor antagonists given frequently during the day.

Rarely, poor symptom relief in a younger patient with a confirmed diagnosis of GORD may be an indication for surgical referral.

Treatment of complications and special groups

Complications resulting from GORD can give rise to additional morbidity or mortality. Resolution of these complications then becomes the aim of treatment. Oesophageal and extra-oesophageal complications may fall into this category.

The aim of treatment is rapid and complete control of reflux to promote healing of tissue damage and resolution of the complication. This can involve use of a proton pump inhibitor and a high dosage is often required (e.g. omeprazole 40 mg daily) until healing or resolution has occurred. Treatment can be continued with a proton pump inhibitor at a lower dose (e.g. omeprazole 20 mg daily). Further management of specific complications is outlined on the opposite page.

Management of complicated GORD		
Complication	**Management**	**Comments**
Benign stricture	Endoscopic dilation using a bougie or inflatable balloon passed over a guidewire. Biopsy and cytology should be done to exclude malignancy. Rarely surgery may be needed	Perforation after dilatation may occur rarely. Signs are persistent chest pain, pain triggered by drinking, fever and surgical emphysema. Management is conservative: fasting, i.v. fluids and antibiotics
Barrett's oesophagus	Treat on basis of symptoms for uncomplicated Barrett's. Complicated Barrett's (dysplasia and ulcer) requires specialist management. Some centres suggest that screening for dysplasia and adenocarcinoma is appropriate every one–two years in young, fit Barrett's patients	Presence of Barrett's ulcer (peptic ulcer within the columnar epithelium) requires treatment with proton pump inhibitors
Haemorrhage or anaemia in elderly patients with oesophagitis	Long-term treatment with a proton-pump inhibitor (colonic cancer must be excluded)	
Respiratory symptoms or reflux	Careful investigation with 24–hour oesophageal pH monitoring should precede treatment	
(i) Recurrent aspiration pneumonia	Anti-reflux surgery is appropriate if patient is fit	
(ii) Nocturnal asthma triggered by reflux	Prop up head of bed, treat reflux symptoms with a proton-pump inhibitor. Optimal medical management of the asthma also required	

Management of GORD in special groups	
Patient group	**Management**
Reflux, dysphagia but no stricture	Dysphagia in this group usually results from oesophagitis. Direct management towards healing oesophagitis rapidly, e.g. proton pump inhibitor
Young patients with incapacitating neurological disease	Severe reflux with oesophageal stricture, ulcer, haemorrhage and pulmonary aspiration common. Treat vigorously with a proton pump inhibitor
Secondary motility disorders (eg. caused by scleroderma or diabetic autonomic neuropathy)	Treat reflux according to severity. Prokinetic agents can be helpful in early scleroderma. Slow gastric emptying may be corrected by cisapride. Anti-reflux surgery (using 'loose-wrap' procedure) may be helpful
Elderly patients with GORD and cardiopulmonary disease	Treat reflux with life-long proton pump inhibition therapy especially if tissue damage is severe
Infants with frequent regurgitation	Will usually resolve with time. May be helped by thickening feeds and nursing in semi-upright seat
Infants with aspiration pneumonia, anaemia, haematemesis and failure to thrive with marked regurgitation	Refer to paediatrician for endoscopy and pH monitoring
Patients on long-term NSAIDs	Increased risk of strictures. Reduce risk by long-term anti-reflux therapy, e.g. long-term proton pump inhibition

7. Prevention of relapse

The size of the problem

The natural history of GORD is characterized by serial relapses and remissions. A minority have almost continuous symptoms — these of course tend to be over-represented in doctors' consulting rooms. Symptomatic relapse occurs in 50–80% of patients within the first 6–12 months after stopping antisecretory treatment. Oesophagitis relapses in 20–80% of individuals six months after stopping treatment. Most studies show relapse rates of between 20 and 35%, with a rate of 80% in patients with particularly severe oesophagitis.

Factors predisposing to early relapse include: severity of oesophagitis; persistence of daytime reflux symptoms at the time of complete healing of oesophagitis; low basal lower oesophageal sphincter pressure; and impaired lower oesophageal motility.

These factors all reflect the severity of the disease; the greater the severity, the more likely the relapse. Relapse is not affected by: age or sex; smoking or alcohol use; disease duration; time taken to heal oesophagitis; or drug used.

There has been some suggestion that patients healed on omeprazole are more likely to relapse, but this is probably because these patients had more severe GORD prior to treatment.

Management of relapse

In a sense, management of GORD is at the point reached for peptic ulcer disease 15 years ago; effective healing is possible in most patients but the majority of cases relapse within a year.

Omeprazole 20 mg daily decreases relapse rate; 65–75% of patients with healed 'refractory oesophagitis' are still in remission after one or two years of continuous treatment.

Low-dose H_2-receptor antagonists are ineffective in preventing the relapse of GORD [17], as is intermittent 'weekend' treatment with omeprazole (20 mg on Friday, Saturday and Sunday each week) [18,19].

Cisapride at doses of 10 mg or 20 mg twice daily or 20 mg at night significantly decreases the relapse rate of symptoms and oesophagitis if taken for 6–12 months after healing with omeprazole or H_2-receptor antagonists. However, the effect is predominantly found in patients with mild (grade I) oesophagitis.

Who needs which maintenance treatment?

Many patients with little or no oesophagitis will enjoy a period of remission after stopping therapy. All patients should, however, be encouraged to persist with the general measures of weight reduction and raising the head of the bed, although it is not proven that these affect the likelihood of relapse.

Intermittent symptomatic relapse, two or three times per year, can be treated with a short course of H_2-receptor antagonists or omeprazole 20 mg daily until symtomatic relief is re-established.

Rapid symptom relapse, if tissue damage is not severe, should be treated with the minimum necessary to maintain adequate symptom relief.

If oesophagitis has never been documented and other measures are ineffective in maintaining remission, the diagnosis of GORD should be confirmed by prolonged oesophageal pH monitoring before embarking on maintenance treatment. In cases when symptoms are severely disruptive and the patient is young, surgery may be an option.

Any patient with severe oesophagitis (grade III and above), particularly if a complication is present (stricture, Barrett's ulcer, haemorrhage), should receive maintenance treatment. Elderly patients should be treated with life-long maintenance omeprazole. The options for younger patients are either life-long omeprazole or anti-reflux surgery.

Appendix I. Epidemiology

A common problem?

Data on disease prevalence are hard to interpret because most rely on surveys based on symptoms and many patients with reflux do not present with classic symptoms (for definition see page 3). An American study of nearly 400 hospital staff found that 29% suffered from heartburn and that 7% experienced it on a daily basis. Similar data have emerged from European studies. However, figures based on typical reflux symptoms alone probably underestimate the true prevalence because one third to one half of all patients with oesophagitis have symptoms not typical for reflux (and presumably others with these symptoms, but no oesophagitis, also have reflux as a cause).

A British general practice survey found that the six-month prevalence of dyspepsia was 38%. Sixty seven percent of these individuals reported heartburn as all or part of their symptoms.

In one North American survey, sufferers from dyspepsia were identified by newspaper advertisement. Ninety five percent of people had reflux-type complaints as part of their symptoms and more than 80% had the presence of GORD confirmed by investigation.

Oesophagitis is the most common lesion found at open-access endoscopy, accounting for approximately 20% of diagnoses. This underestimates the number of individuals with symptomatic reflux because, at least among patients referred to hospitals, endoscopic oesophagitis is only found in 60% of those with classic reflux symptoms.

Clearly, reflux is a very common problem. Many sufferers do not consult doctors and an even smaller proportion are referred to hospital — hence the concept of the 'GORD iceberg' popularized by Castell.

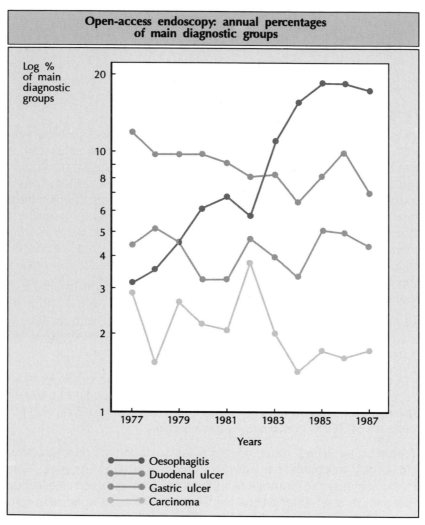

Annual percentages of main diagnostic groups in an open access endoscopy service. Published by permission from Gear MWL and Wilkinson SP, Br J Hosp Med 1989, 41:38–44.

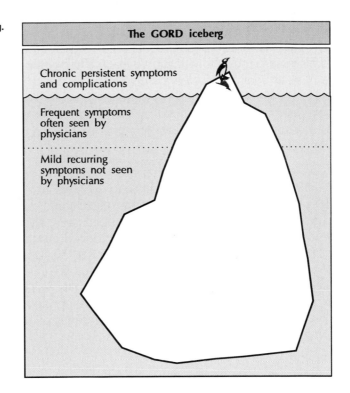

The GORD iceberg.
Adapted by
permission of
DO Castell.
Grad Hospital,
Philadelphia,
PA, USA.

The GORD iceberg

Chronic persistent symptoms
and complications

Frequent symptoms
often seen by
physicians

Mild recurring
symptoms not seen
by physicians

AI. EPIDEMIOLOGY

What kind of person develops GORD?

GORD is probably a disorder of the Western world; it appears to be uncommon in Africa and the Far East. The incidence of endoscopic oesophagitis is highest in people aged between sixty and seventy years and is more common in men than women. The same is true for the complications of oesophageal stricture and Barrett's oesophagus, which together comprise about 20% of patients with endoscopic oeso-phagitis.

These observations may not reflect the whole spectrum of GORD for which no data are available. However, if the dyspeptic population as a whole is any guide, symptoms are slightly more common in the under 40s and show little sex preponderance.

Associations of reflux with pregnancy, obesity and smoking are well recognized. Less widely appreciated is the association between eden-tulousness and benign stricture in patients with GORD.

Natural history of GORD

Symptomatic gastro-oesophageal reflux is a disorder of relapses and remissions in most individuals, although a few patients suffer continual relapse as soon as treatment is discontinued. There is little evidence to support the notion that patients with a long history of symptoms develop severe complications. Indeed, up to 25% of patients with benign stricture secondary to gastro-oesophageal reflux have few, or no antecedent reflux symptoms [20].

Long-term (20-year) follow-up of many patients with 'hiatus hernia' in the 1960s found that symptomatic improvement with time was common [21]. However, it is unclear whether all patients had GORD (as discussed previously) and recent follow-up studies (although shorter term — three to four years) of better characterized groups of patients tell a different story. In one report, symptoms had disappeared in only 15% of patients (on or off treatment) over a three-year period. The findings are independent of whether or not oesophagitis was present at the start of treatment. Interestingly, endoscopic oesophagitis may appear or disappear during follow-up quite independently of the course of symptoms [22,23].

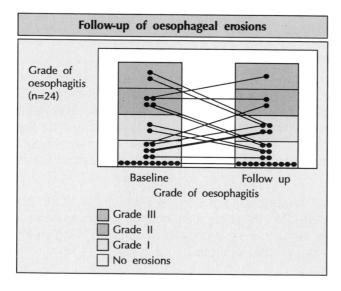

Follow-up of oesophageal erosions

Grade of oesophagitis (n=24)

Baseline   Follow up
Grade of oesophagitis

☐ Grade III
☐ Grade II
☐ Grade I
☐ No erosions

Changes in grade of oesophagitis over a mean 40 month follow-up period in 24 patients — new erosions developed in some people while in others the oesophagitis healed. Published by permission from Schindlbeck NE, *et al.* Gut 1992, 33: 1016–1019.

Appendix II. Pathophysiology

The essential features of GORD result from disordered function of distal oesophageal and gastric smooth muscle. Vagal nerve damage may underlie some of these abnormalities. Disordered anatomy around the diaphragmatic hiatus is an important contributory factor. Minor degrees of reflux during the day, especially after meals, are normal although this is exaggerated in reflux patients and can often occur at night.

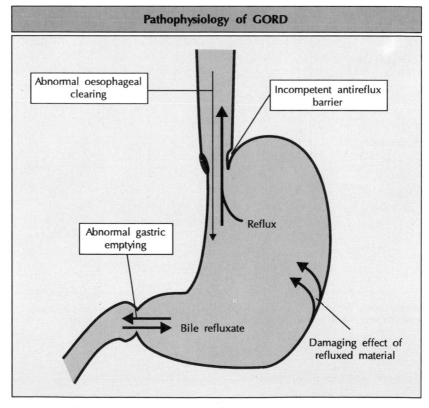

Pathophysiology of GORD

Abnormal oesophageal clearing

Incompetent antireflux barrier

Reflux

Abnormal gastric emptying

Bile refluxate

Damaging effect of refluxed material

A summary of the chief pathogenic factors involved in gastro-oesophageal reflux disease.

Failure of the reflux barrier

- Reflux usually occurs during brief relaxations of the lower oesophageal sphincter; many such relaxations occur after a 'failed swallow' or are initiated by gastric distension. These occur in normal individuals but are more frequent and more often associated with reflux in patients with GORD.

- Other mechanisms include reflux across a low-pressure sphincter (especially patients with more severe oesophagitis) and reflux provoked by straining and coughing (particularly in patients with airways obstruction).

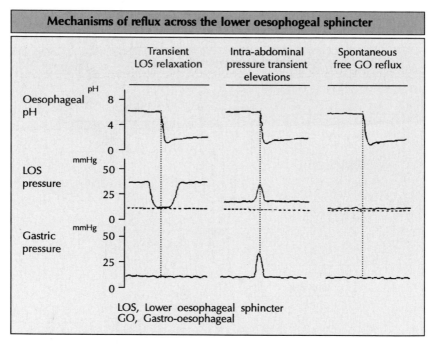

Mechanisms of reflux across the lower oesophogeal sphincter

LOS, Lower oesophageal sphincter
GO, Gastro-oesophageal

Mechanisms of reflux across the lower oesophageal sphincter. Reprinted with permission from The New England Journal of Medicine. Dodds WJ, *et al.* 1982, 307:1547–1552.

- Drugs such as anticholinergic agents, nitrates, calcium antagonists and theophylline derivatives decrease lower oesophageal sphincter pressure, prompting reflux. Nicotine and caffeine have similar effects.

- The diaphragmatic crus which normally surrounds the lower oesophageal sphincter (as the oesophagus passes through the diaphragm from the thorax to the abdomen) acts as an 'external sphincter', especially to prevent reflux during straining. Failure of the crus closing mechanism may occur and contribute to reflux.

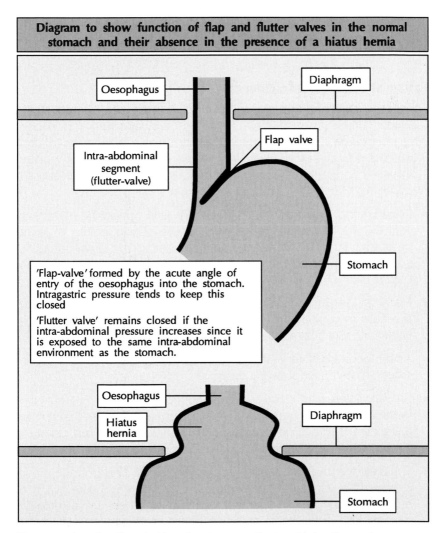

Diagram to show function of flap and flutter valves in the normal stomach and their absence in the presence of a hiatus hernia

Oesophagus

Diaphragm

Flap valve

Intra-abdominal segment (flutter-valve)

Stomach

'Flap-valve' formed by the acute angle of entry of the oesophagus into the stomach. Intragastric pressure tends to keep this closed

'Flutter valve' remains closed if the intra-abdominal pressure increases since it is exposed to the same intra-abdominal environment as the stomach.

Oesophagus

Hiatus hernia

Diaphragm

Stomach

Diagram to show the effect of a hiatus hernia on oesophagogastric junction anatomy.

AII. PATHOPHYSIOLOGY

- Hiatus hernia, although common in asymptomatic individuals over the age of 50 years, is present in 90% of patients with oesophagitis. It seems to contribute by providing a small reservoir of gastric contents easily available for reflux when the lower oesophageal sphincter relaxes.

The presence of a hiatus hernia also counteracts the protective effect of other mechanical factors which normally help prevent reflux; these include the 'flap valve', caused by the acute angle of entry of the oesophagus into the stomach, and the 'flutter valve' effect of the intra-abdominal oesophageal segment.

Failure of oesophageal clearance

Clearance of oesophageal content depends on efficient peristaltic function ('primary peristalsis' — initiated by swallowing and 'secondary peristalsis' — an evolutionary response to oesophageal distension) and secretion of saliva. Primary peristalsis is more important because this results in swallowing of alkaline saliva which offers a neutralizing effect.

- Distal oesophageal peristalsis is abnormal in up to 50% of patients with GORD, especially those with severe oesophagitis. Impaired peristalsis is not corrected by medical healing of the oesophagitis, suggesting that it is a primary phenomenon and not simply secondary to oesophageal wall inflammation.

- Many of the drugs which decrease lower oesophageal sphincter pressure (see page 44) also impair distal oesophageal peristalsis. Heavy alcohol intake may have similar effects.

- Acid clearance is very slow if the secretion of saliva is inhibited, for example, by anticholinergic drugs.

- Salivary flow is stimulated by acid-induced heartburn ('waterbrash'). In patients with the most severe oesophagitis (e.g. those with strictures and Barrett's oesophagus) this reflex is impaired because oesophageal sensitivity to acid is decreased or absent.

- The oesophagus is in 'double jeopardy' at night: oesophageal clearance is less efficient in the recumbent position and swallowing of acid-neutralizing saliva does not occur during sleep. Transient lower oesophageal sphincter relaxation (and thus reflux) is fortunately rare during the night but becomes more common as reflux disease progresses. For these reasons, even a single reflux episode can lead to prolonged exposure of the oesophageal mucosa to acid. This may increase symptoms during the day by sensitizing the oesophageal pain receptors or may incréase tissue damage.

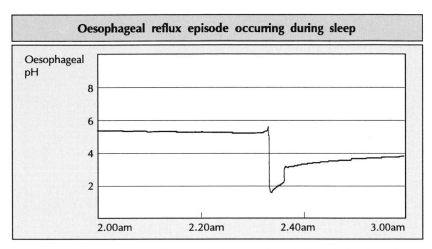

Reflux episode occurring during sleep recorded by oesophageal pH monitoring. Note the long period before the the intraoesophageal pH reaches 4.

Gastric factors

- Delayed gastric emptying is found in up to 40% of patients with GORD. This could promote reflux either by extending the time after meals during which gastric contents are available for reflux or by promoting transient lower oesophageal sphincter relaxation through gastric distension.

- Acid and pepsin are of primary importance. 'No acid, no ulcer' is as true for GORD as it is for peptic ulcer disease. Alkaline reflux (reflux of unacidified small bowel contents) occurs rarely, if at all, except in patients with pernicious anaemia or following total gastrectomy.

- Curiously, in contrast with duodenal ulcer disease, gastric acid output is not increased in most patients with a hiatus hernia. Exceptions are patients with the very rare Zollinger–Ellison syndrome and some patients with severe oesophageal damage, who may have increased basal gastric acid output.

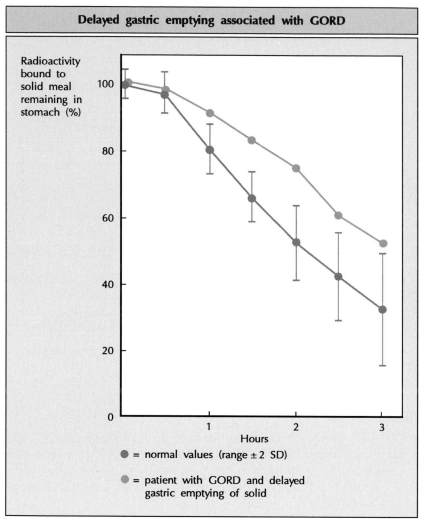

Delayed emptying of a radiolabelled solid meal in a patient with GORD compared to a control measurement.

- Duodenogastric reflux allows bile, which can damage the oesophagus if refluxed (albeit mildly on its own), to be present in gastric juice. It is not clear whether this process, which occurs in healthy individuals, is increased in reflux disease but its contribution is minor compared with that of acid and pepsin.

Acid secretion in GORD compared with controls and patients with duodenal ulceration. Published by permission from Williams CB, *et al.* Lancet 1967, i:184–185. © The Lancet, 1967.

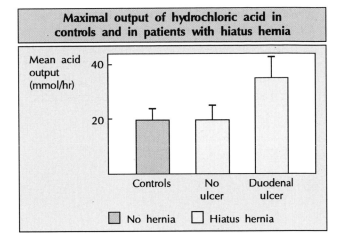

AII. PATHOPHYSIOLOGY

Factors influencing the development of oesophagitis

- Patients with oesophagitis have, on average, more acid reflux than those without. People with the most severe complications tend to have the most acid reflux. Acid-peptic damage to the oesophagus is cumulative over a 24 hour period; more acid exposure leads to more mucosal damage. There is good evidence to support the notion that Barrett's oesophagus results from healing of ulcerative oesophagitis by columnar metaplastic epithelium.

- As acid reflux increases, a progressively larger proportion of the total acid exposure occurs during the night because of an increase in reflux episodes and delayed clearance of refluxed gastric contents. However, reflux is damaging whenever it occurs and it seems unwise to emphasize an intrinsically greater damaging effect from night-time rather than daytime reflux.

- Factors determining mucosal resistance to acid-peptic attack (such as tight intercellular junctions, cell membrane channels for expelling hydrogen ions and mucus secretion) are only beginning to be understood and it is not clear whether individuals destined to develop oesophagitis have impaired defences.

- Some drugs, particularly NSAIDs, tetracycline and slow release potassium preparations, can cause oesophageal ulceration and stricture in their own right. NSAIDs have also been implicated in the development of strictures in patients with GORD.

- There is no evidence that *Helicobacter pylori* infection contributes to the development of oesophagitis, although the organism may colonize any metaplastic columnar epithelium. It is uncertain whether the infection contributes to the development of Barrett's ulcers (peptic ulcer within the columnar metaplastic gastric epithelium abnormally present above the lower oesophageal sphincter).

Appendix III. Investigations

Different tests define different aspects of GORD and are thus, in many respects, complementary. The choice of test will depend on the question to be addressed. Some investigations detect mucosal damage (air-contrast radiology, endoscopy), others mucosal acid sensitivity (acid perfusion test, prolonged pH monitoring) and yet others gastro-oesophageal reflux (radiology, pH monitoring, scintigraphy). Because reflux is intermittent it is not surprising that prolonged tests, for example, 12 or 24 hour oesophageal pH monitoring, are most sensitive for the detection of acid reflux.

Investigations for GORD	
Radiography	
Barium swallow	A widely available important first step which can show functional and anatomical abnormalities in patients with heartburn or dysphagia (see figure on page 52). Most important to detect strictures in patients with dysphagia. Better than endoscopy for some lesions, e.g. rings and webs.
Double-contrast radiograph	Detects subtle mucosal abnormalities suggestive of oesophagitis.
Endoscopy	Most sensitive method for assessing tissue damage. Severity of macroscopic oesophagitis can be graded by endoscopic appearance. Most popular system is the Savary–Miller system (see table on page 53). Biopsy and cytology capability important. Barrett's oesophagus is most easily diagnosed at endoscopy.
Acid perfusion	If available, a simple, useful test for mucosal acid sensitivity. Comparison of symptoms made on perfusion through a naso-oesophageal tube with 0.1N HCl and N saline. Positive test is reproduction of typical symptoms on perfusion with acid but not saline. Sensitivity and specificity ~80% for acid-induced pain.

continued

Investigations for GORD (continued)	
24–hour oesophageal pH monitoring	Most sensitive and specific investigation for acid reflux. Can be done as an outpatient procedure and is most helpful if performed during the patients normal activities. Allows quantitation of acid reflux and correlation of symptoms with events (see figures on pages 55–57) > 7% of total monitoring period at oesophageal pH < 4 = excessive reflux.
Gastro-oesophageal scintigraphy	Gastro–oesophageal reflux of a radioisotope is measured. No more sensitive than barium radiography. Not widely available.
Short-term pH monitoring	Examples are 3-hour post-prandial monitoring and the standard acid reflux test (SART). Less sensitive than prolonged pH monitoring and does not allow symptom–reflux correlation. Not widely done in UK.
Oesophageal pressure monitoring	Can detect abnormal oesophageal motility or low basal LOS pressure. Does not diagnose GORD, but could be helpful in other conditions, e.g. achalasia, diffuse oesophageal spasm. Can now be done at the same time as the 24-hour pH test.
Acid clearance test	Measures the number of swallows required to clear an exogenous acid load from the distal oesophagus. Of little diagnostic value.

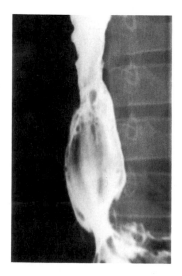

Benign stricture caused by proven reflux in a child; this patient subsequently underwent fundoplication. Published by permission of AD Taylor, Hull Royal Infirmary, UK.

Savary Millar Grading System of oesophagitis	
Grade I	Red streaks, erosions, non-confluent
Grade II	Confluent erosions, not circumferential
Grade III	Circumferential erosions
Grade IV	Stricture/Barrett's oesophagus

AIII. INVESTIGATIONS

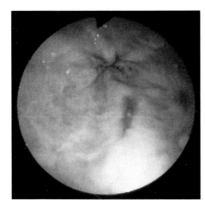

**Savary Miller grade I oesophagitis.
Single longitudinal erosion in distal
oesophagus.***

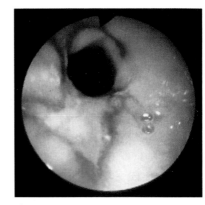

**Savary Miller grade II oesophagitis.
Confluent non-circumferential erosions.***

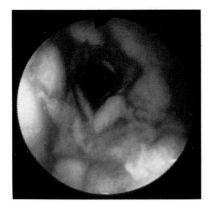

**Savary Miller grade III oesophagitis.
Circumferential oesophageal erosions.***

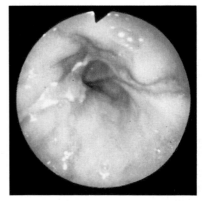

**Savary Miller grade IV oesophagitis.
Benign stricture.***

*Published by permission of GNJ Tytgat, Academic Medical Centre, Amsterdam, The Nether-
lands. © Astra 1993.

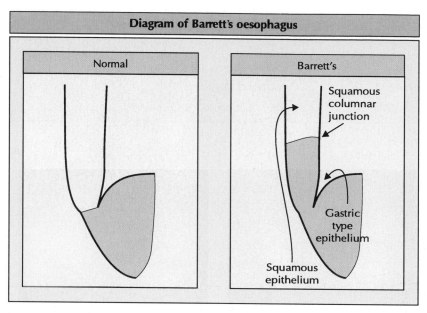

Diagram of Barrett's oesophagus.

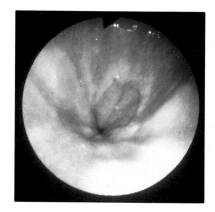

Normal oesophagus with normal squamo-columnar junction.*

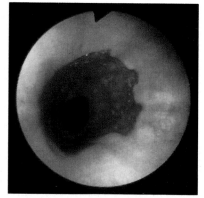

Savary Miller grade IV oesophagitis. Columnar lined Barrett's oesophagus.*

An oesophageal biopsy showing gross elongation of the papillae. There is a minor degree of basal cell hyperplasia and scattered inflammatory cells in the epithelium (Haematoxylin eosin). Published by permission of A Price, Northwick Park Hospital, Harrow, UK.

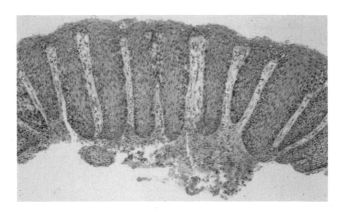

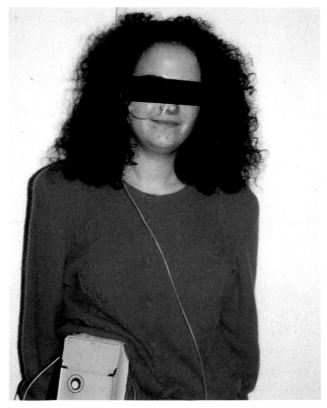

Slide showing patient with a pH electrode *in situ* connected to a portable recorder.

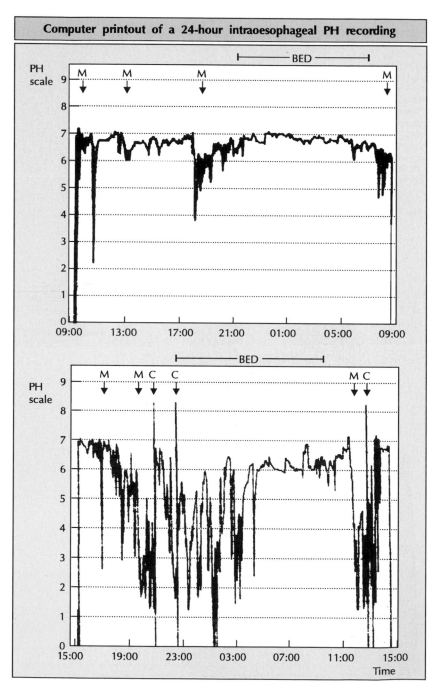

Computer printout of a 24-hour intraoesophageal PH recording

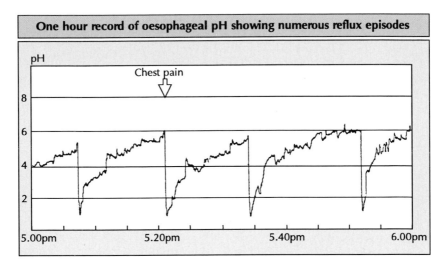

One hour record of oesophageal pH showing numerous reflux episodes

Coincidence of a reflux episode and chest pain (time recorded by patient on a diary card).

Facing page: Computer printout of a 24-hour intraoesophageal pH recording showing normal amounts of reflux occurring mainly after meals (M) (upper trace). Lower trace shows abnormal amounts of reflux occurring in GORD; note the frequent nocturnal episodes (C = chest pain).

References

1. Klinkenberg-Knol EC, Meuwissen SGM: **Combined gastric and oesophageal 24-hour pH monitoring and oesophageal manometry in patients with reflux disease resistant to treatment with omeprazole.** *Aliment Pharmacol Therap* 1990, **4**:485–495.

2. Alban Davies H, Jones DB, Rhodes J: **'Esophageal angina' as the cause of chest pain.** *JAMA* 1982, **248**:2274–2278.

3. Sontag S, O'Connell S, Khandelwal S, *et al.*: **Most asthmatics have gastroesophageal reflux with or without bronchodilator therapy.** *Gastroenterology* 1990, **99**:613–620.

4. Flook D, Soddard CJ: **Gastro-oesophageal reflux and oesophagitis before and after vagotomy for duodenal ulcer.** *Br J Surg* 1985, **72**:804–807.

5. Graham DY, Lacey Smith J, Patterson DJ: **Why do apparently healthy people use antacid tablets?** *Am J Gastroenterol* 1983, **78**:257–260.

6. Scarpignato C, Galmiche JP: **Antacids and alginates in the treatment of gastro-oesophageal reflux disease: How do they work and how much are they clinically useful?** In *Advances in Drug Therapy of Gastro-oesophageal Reflux Disease. Frontiers of Gastrointestinal Research* Vol 20 edited by Scarpignato C. Karger:Basel pp 153–181.

7. Bate CM, Keeling PWN, O'Morrain C, *et al.*: **Comparison of omeprazole and cimetidine in reflux oesophagitis; symptomatic, endoscopic, and histological evaluations.** *Gut* 1990, **31**:968–972.

8. Sandmark S, Carlsson R, Fausa O, *et al:* **Omeprazole or ranitidine in treatment of reflux esophagitis. Results of a double-blind, randomized, Scandinavian multicenter study.** *Scand J Gastroenterol* 1988, **23**:625–632.

9. Lundell L, Backman L, Ekstrom P, *et al.*: **Omeprazole or high-dose ranitidine in the treatment of patients with reflux oesophagitis not responding to 'standard doses' of H_2-receptor antagonists.** *Aliment Pharmacol Ther* 1990, **4**:145–155.

10. Hungin APS, Gunn AD, Bate CM, *et al.*: **A comparison of the efficacy of omeprazole 20mg once daily with ranitidine 150 mg bd in the relief of symptomatic disease in general practice.** *Br J Clin Res* 1993, **4**:73–88.

11. Smith PM, Kerr GD, Cockel R, *et al.*: **A comparison of omeprazole and ranitidine in the prevention of recurrence of oesophageal stricture.** *Gut* 1993, **34** (suppl 4):S19.

12. Toussaint J, Gossuin A, Deruyttere M, *et al.*: **Healing and prevention of relapse of reflux oesophagitis by cisapride.** *Gut* 1991, **32**:1280–1285.

13. Tytgat GNJ, Anker Hansen OJ, Carling L, *et al.*: **Effect of cisapride on relapse of reflux oesophagitis healed with an antisecretory drug.** *Scand J Gastroenterol* 1992, **27**:175–183.

REFERENCES

14. Hillman AL, Bloom BS, Fendrick M, et al.: **Cost and quality effects of alternative treatments for persistent gastroesophageal disease.** Arch Intern Invest 1992, **152**:1467–1472.

15. Bate CM: **Cost effectiveness of omeprazole in the treatment of reflux oesophagitis.** BrJ Med Economics 1991, **1**:53–61.

16. Bate CM, Richardson PDI: **Symptomatic assessment and cost effectiveness of treatments for reflux oesophagitis: comparisons of omeprazole and histamine H₂-receptor antagonists.** Br J Med Economics 1992, **2**:37–48.

17. Bianchi Porro G, Pace F, Sangaletti O, et al.: **High dose famotidine in the maintenance treatment of refractory esophagitis: Results of a 'medium term' open study.** Am J Gastroenterol 1991, **86**:1585–1587.

18. Zietun P, Isal JP, Barbier P: **Comparison of two dosage regimens of omeprazole – 10mg once daily and 20 mg weekends – as prophylaxis against recurrence of reflux oesophagitis.** World Congress of Gastroenterology Sydney, Australia, 1990 p58.

19. Dent J, Mackinnon M, Reed W, et al.: **Omeprazole prevents relapse of peptic oesophagitis.** World Congress of Gastroenterology Sydney, Australia, 1990 p4.

20. Patterson DJ, Graham DY, Lacey Smith J, et al.: **Natural history of benign oesophageal stricture treated by dilatation.** Gastroenterology 1983, **85**:346–350.

21. Palmer ED: **The hiatus hernia-esophagitis-esophageal stricture complex: a twenty year prospective study.** Am J Med 1968, **44**:566–579.

22. Pace F, Santalucia F, Bianchi Porro G, et al.: **Natural history of gastro-oesophageal reflux disease without oesophagitis.** Gut 1991, **32**:845–848.

23. Schindlbeck NE, Klauser AG, Berghammer G, et al.: **Three year follow-up of patients with gastro-oesophageal reflux disease.** Gut 1992, **33**:1016–1019.